Infused Water

Infused water benefits, and delicious infused water recipes!

Table of Contents

Introduction iv

Chapter 1 - Things you Need to Know About Fruit Infused Water 6

Chapter 2 - Benefits of Fruit Infused Water 15

Chapter 3 - Detox Fruit Infused Water Recipes .. 20

Chapter 4 - Invigorating and Hydrating Water Recipes 26

Chapter 5 - Weight Loss Aid Recipes 31

Conclusion 36

Introduction

I want to thank you and congratulate you for downloading the book, *"Infused Water: Infused water benefits, and delicious infused water recipes!"*

This book contains helpful information about infused water, and all of its benefits.

Everyone needs adequate amounts of water to survive. Civilizations are known to spring from where clean water abounds. Clean and potable water sources are also essential requirements before modern communities are built. Even still, a lot of people opt to drink flavored drinks. These drinks can do your body more harm than good. A healthier and more refreshing option is infused water.

This book will explain to you tips and techniques that will allow you to successfully create your own delicious infused water from home.

This book provides a range of recipes that will assist in detoxifying your body, keeping you hydrated, and will help you lose weight! Not only do you get these benefits, but the recipes are also delicious, and easy to make!

With these recipes, it will be easier for you to make the healthy switch in your drink of choice.

Thanks again for downloading this book, I hope you enjoy it!

Chapter 1 - Things you Need to Know About Fruit Infused Water

The body is 60% water, and as a result needs a constant supply of water to function well. Water helps your body flush out toxins and cleanses your organs. Health experts recommend consuming at least 8 glasses of water each day to provide the hydration that your body needs. Drinking this amount can also help keep harmful substances out of your system, and can even assist in weight loss.

Not all people have the same ideal amount of water intake. The minimum intake of water should be eight glasses and above. Drinking the amount below the suggested mark may not give you the full benefits of drinking water. Sadly, not everyone is fond of drinking water.

Most prefer drinking something with flavor such as soda, packed juice, or other sugary drinks. Consuming too much sugar can harm your body and the drinks that most people prefer over water contain large amounts of sugar. Even the commercially produced flavored water contains high amount of sugar.

If you want to drink something with flavor, then fruit infused water is the one to choose. It has no added sugar, but can have plenty of flavor with the right amount fruits. You can use different fruits to make your water sour or sweet, depending on what drinks you prefer. The idea is to make the fruit infused water yourself, so you can be certain that you will be drinking something that is chemical-free, fresh, affordable, and without added sugar.

It is not difficult to make your own fruit flavored water and you can store your remaining water in the refrigerator and drink it later. Make it a family habit to drink fruit infused water for a fit, healthier, and more beautiful body.

Determining the Right Amount of Water Consumption for Your Weight

The required amount of water that you need to drink a day is eight glasses minimum. For children, at least six glasses of water per day is recommended.

However, the ideal amount of water to drink varies from one individual to the other. If you weigh more, then you need to drink more water in order to help your body achieve a fit and healthy state.

There is a formula to help you determine your ideal water intake. Take note that "lbs" is your weight in pounds and "oz" is the amount of water you need to take in ounces.

To get your ideal water consumption and gain the most benefits, use this formula:

$$lbs \div 2 = oz$$

To get the number of glasses you need to drink, use this formula:

oz ÷ 8 = the number of glasses of water you need consume per day

A regular drinking glass contains eight ounces of liquid, which is why you need to divide the number of ounces you need to take by eight. Counting the number of glasses is easier than monitoring the volume by ounce.

For example, if you are someone who weighs 180 lbs, then follow the given formula to get your ideal water intake:

$$180 \text{ lbs} \div 2 = 90 \text{ oz}$$

You need to consume this many glasses of water per day:

$$90 \text{ oz} \div 8 = 11.25 \text{ or } 12 \text{ glasses per day}$$

It is better to always round off the answer to the next whole number to maximize your water intake. You can always go beyond your ideal water intake. Once you have discovered what infused water recipes you like, you will want to drink more water than ever before.

To make your fruit infused water more flavorful, you can add herbs or vegetables or both – it really depends on your preferences. Over time you will adjust the taste of different recipes, and discover more combinations that you can try.

The Things You Need for Your Fruit Infused Water

Contrary to what some people think, preparing fruit infused water is not complicated and it is not expensive. You only need to use everyday tools and things that can be found in your kitchen.

Choose Organic and Fresh Ingredients

In choosing your ingredients (be it fruit, herb, or vegetable), you need to make sure to choose fresh and organic produce to get the maximum benefits. It is best if you can grow your own ingredients, because this way you can be certain that you are using chemical-free ingredients.

You can choose any fruit, but it is best to start with fruits that provide more juice. Choose fruits that are ripe enough to release their best flavor in the water, giving it just the right amount of sweetness. If you choose any of the citrus fruits, then you may need to add a sweet fruit to counter the sourness. It is an absolute no-no to add sugar to your flavored water, but if it can't be helped, then choose stevia to sweeten your water a bit. Remember that you still need to teach yourself to appreciate the natural sweetness that the fruits provide and eliminate stevia later on. Do not use overripe produce in making your fruit infused water.

There are some fruit infused water drinkers who like adding mint to their water to make it more refreshing. You can choose to add or not to add some herbs. You will find recipes in this book that call for herb addition to make the flavor more intense. Herbs complement most fruits and vegetables when infused in water. You can conduct an experiment and see which herb you prefer to go with a certain fruit or vegetable before making a large batch of infused water.

Water to Use

You can use purified, filtered, or tap water – you can choose any type of water as long as it is to your liking. You can also choose sparkling water if you want added fizz in your drink.

Muddler

A muddler is usually a wooden spoon that you can use to slightly mash or bruise your ingredients and help you release the flavor in the water. Don't expect to get the flavor that you desire by just soaking your ingredients without doing anything. You need to muddle your ingredients to get the right mingling of flavors in your water.

Pitcher and Jar

It is recommended to prepare your fruit infused water in large batches. You can use a two-quart pitcher or a Mason jar. Preparing your fruit infused water in big batches is handy, because you will always have ready-to-drink flavored water ready to go. It can also make you drink more often when you see the prepared infused water in your refrigerator.

Different Fruit Infusion Water Bottle

You may or may not choose to own a fruit infusion bottle, but these are handy to have, especially if you travel a lot. Bringing your own fruit infused water can prevent you from buying beverages that have a high sugar content. It is also more practical if you have your own fruit infused water wherever you go.

Other Things You May Need

There is no other special equipment required for making infused water. Your standard kitchen equipment like your knife, chopping board, some plates, trays, and apron are all you need for preparing your fruit infused water. In some cases, you will also need a strainer or sieve with fine mesh.

Important Facts about Fruit Infused Water

Before getting started, here are some fruit infused water facts to keep in mind:

Different Methods of Infusing Water

There are different methods of infusing your water, but most recipes in this book use only one method because it can make the water more flavorful in a more convenient manner.

The first method is soaking. You just have to peel your ingredients, chop them a little or slice them, and then let them soak in water. Let it sit in your refrigerator for two to eight hours before drinking. This method may be the simplest among the methods but the flavor you will get is not as intense as the other methods.

The second method is pureeing your ingredients. You will need to use a strainer or sieve when doing this method. After you have pureed your ingredients place the puree in your pitcher and pour your cold water over it. Let it sit for a while to allow the flavors to distribute before pouring some in your glass. This method is a bit tedious, but will provide a stronger flavor.

The third method is the widely used method in all recipes in this book. After preparing your ingredients, you need to layer them at the bottom of your pitcher or jar. Mash them a little to release the flavor then add ice and water. Stir for a bit and let it sit in your refrigerator for at least four hours before serving.

The Best Length of Time to Infuse

It is advisable to infuse your water for at least an hour at room temperature and for two to four hours in the refrigerator before drinking. There are some who prefer their flavored water to sit in the refrigerator overnight.

Number of Times you can Refill your Pitcher

You can refill your pitcher of fruit infused water up to three to six times especially if you have guests in the house. Make sure to refill when the pitcher is half empty to redistribute the flavors and have only a subtle change in the intensity of flavor. Adding too much water can make it go bland. Muddle it for a bit to release some more flavor before serving it to your guests.

The Bitter Taste in Your Flavored Water

The rind of most fruits, especially citrus, gives fruit infused water its splendid aroma. The peelings are also packed with vitamins and nutrients that can make your fruit infused water more beneficial. The only catch is that the peelings can make your fruit infused water bitter. If you love the scent, but hate the bitter taste, then let the peelings stay in the water for only four hours. If you think you might not be able to take them out within that period, then it is best if you peel off your fruit first before infusing your water. It is recommended not to let your ingredients stay in the water for more than 24 hours, even if you put your pitcher in the refrigerator. Also, you need to discard your fruit infused water immediately if it starts to have a foul smell or turns a different color. Don't try tasting it because there is a good chance that bacteria and other microorganisms have already made their way into your drink.

Hot or Cold

It is true that pouring hot water over your ingredients may produce faster results in terms of extracting flavors. Hot water, however, can destroy the important nutrients that your ingredients contain. You will not gain extra benefits that the flavored water can give. One suggestion is to let your ingredients sit at room temperature (do not use cold water) for at least an hour and not more than four hours before adding some ice or before putting it in your refrigerator.

Eating the Fruits in Your Fruit Infused Water

There is no rule that forbids you to eat the fruits in your fruit infused water. It is a different story if you still need to refill your pitcher. You won't be able to achieve the same flavor intensity as the first serving if you have less fruits in your pitcher during refill. You can, however, eat the excess fruits that you will no longer need from your fruit infused water. You can also garnish your glass with the remaining fruits if you like or add them to your dish.

Chapter 2 - Benefits of Fruit Infused Water

Fresh fruit juices are healthy, but they also contain large amounts of sugar which can harm your body. If you want to drink something healthy and with flavor, then choose fruit infused water.

Keeps the Body Well Hydrated

Water can help to distribute nutrients through the entire body. It also aids in circulation and digestion. It can help you keep your body well hydrated and avoid being thirsty. A person feels thirsty when his or her body's fluid level becomes low. When a person's body does not get the right amount of fluids, their concentration and focus gets compromised.

If your body is dehydrated, then there is a huge possibility of experiencing joint pains, headaches, and indigestion. To avoid these from happening, it is advisable to keep your body well hydrated all the time and drink water immediately when thirst sets in.

Healthier Alternative to Sugary Drinks

You may think that energy drinks and fruit juices are healthy for you because of the energy boost that they provide. However, this boost actually comes from the sugar rush from these drinks. What happens after your sugar rush is not good for the body. Infused water gives you the flavor and energy boost without the sugar rush. Instead, you get healthy nutrients that nourish the body.

Helps Curb your Appetite

Fruit infused water has the ability to curb your appetite, and makes you feel more satiated. This forces you to eat the necessary amount of food that your body needs and nothing more. Due to this reason, fruit infused water can help you keep the extra weight off and it can help you regulate your blood sugar. It also helps prevent heartburn.

Aids in Weight Loss

If you are someone who has been struggling with weight issues for quite some time now, then you can turn to fruit infused water to help you lose weight. It is a known fact that drinking lots of water can help you lose weight because it can flush out the toxins and make you feel full for a long time. The beauty of drinking fruit infused water is that you also gain added nutrients from the fruits that can help you keep the excess pounds off.

It's Good for the Whole Family

Even kids can drink fruit infused water, and it's great to teach your younger children to get used to drinking fruit infused water over soda or other sugary beverages. Getting them started on this healthy drinking habit early will allow them to carry on such a practice as they move to adulthood.

Fruit Infused Water can Help Energize the Muscles

Your cells will degenerate if they do not get enough liquids. This can lead to muscle fatigue. The cells of your muscles need liquids to function properly. Before exercising and in between exercises, it is a good practice to drink some fruit infused water. Drinking fruit infused water during workouts can help keep your body stay hydrated despite the physical exertion and sweating.

Helps Improve your Immune System

Citrus infused water, in particular, can boost your body's nutrient absorbing capacity. The citrus family is rich in vitamin C which is known for enhancing the immune system. The more you drink fruit infused water, the better it is for your health.

It is Economical

The cost of preparing your own fruit infused water is lower than buying bottled or canned beverages from your local grocery stores. You can use the same ingredients by refilling your pitcher up to six times within a period of 24 hours. You can store the infused water in your refrigerator for up to three days without the ingredients.

Fruit Infused Water Helps Reduce the Risk of Certain Cancers

There are cancers that develop from unhealthy digestive systems. Studies have revealed that drinking enough water can dilute the cancer causing agents that invade the body. These agents are flushed out of the body so they cannot cause any harm. The added nutrients provided by the fruits can help in making the body strong and healthy so it can fight harmful invaders.

Wear Radiantly Beautiful and Youthful Looking Skin

Dehydration can also affect the health of your skin – it can make your skin look old, dry, and wrinkled. To keep your skin glowing and well hydrated, you should drink fruit infused water. The extra vitamins, minerals, and other nutrients that the ingredients provide in your infused water can help make your skin look younger than your actual age, and more radiant as well. It is recommended to try drinking citrus fruit infused water because the citrus family can provide the most effective benefits for achieving great looking skin.

It Helps Prevent Constipation

If you are someone who experiences constipation often, there is a good chance that it's because you aren't drinking enough water. For a lot of people, drinking water is not appealing because it's tasteless. Fruit infused water can help solve that dilemma because it's packed with flavors. It also comes in thousands of fruit, herb, and vegetable combinations to choose from. You don't need to force yourself to drink plain water to end your constipation problem. You can choose to drink the flavorful fruit infused water instead.

Chapter 3 - Detox Fruit Infused Water Recipes

The recipes for fruit infused water in this chapter have detoxifying properties that can help you cleanse your body, and make sure it stays in good condition.

Ultimate Detox Drink

This recipe has lemon, cucumber, and parsley that are famous for their detoxifying properties. These ingredients help to clean your body from the inside and out.

You will need:

1 small to medium sized cucumber

2 lemons

1 medium sized bunch of parsley

1/2 cup cranberries (for added flavor)

1 small sized bunch of cilantro

2 quarts water

2 cups crushed ice

Here's how:

You need to peel your ingredients first to avoid getting a bitter taste. You can keep the peelings on your lemon but don't let it sit in your water for more than four hours. Keeping the peelings can give your fruit infused water a marvelous aroma, but keeping it in the water for more than four hours can make your fruit infused water bitter. Remove the stems of your herbs.

Slice your fruits and chop your herbs a bit (don't crush them). Line your ingredients at the bottom of your pitcher. Muddle a little, then add ice and water. Infuse for at least four hours in the refrigerator before serving. You can also squeeze a bit of your lemon in the water to make the flavor more intense.

You can refill your pitcher once it's half empty to get almost the same intensity of flavors. You can use the same ingredients in your pitcher four to five times within the day.

Minty Gooseberry Infused Water

If you want to try something new and refreshing, then you've got to try this detox water recipe.

You will need:

7 to 10 gooseberries

1 lemon

2 sprigs of mint

1/2 tsp salt

2 quarts water

1 cup crushed ice

Here's how:

Cut your lemon in half and get at least half teaspoon of lemon zest from the half of lemon. Remove the seeds from your gooseberries then scoop the flesh out. Place your lemon zest and gooseberries in the pitcher and add the salt before adding some water. Crush the mint leaves and add them to the water. Slice the other lemon half and put the lemon slices in the water.

Muddle for a bit then add ice and the remaining water. Infuse for at least four hours in the refrigerator. Strain, serve, and enjoy.

Melon and Cucumber Galore

Summer is never complete without tasting the delightful combination of melon and cucumber plus some more.

You will need:

1 small sized cucumber

1/2 honeydew

1/4 watermelon

1/4 cantaloupe

2 quarts water

1 to 2 cups crushed ice

Here's how:

Wash your ingredients and drain the excess water. Peel your fruits. Cut your cucumber into thin slices. Cut your honeydew, watermelon, and cantaloupe into large cube chunks. Line your ingredients at the bottom of your pitcher and muddle for a bit. Add ice and 2 quarts water. Infuse for at least four hours in the refrigerator before serving.

You can refill your pitcher when it is half empty up to four times within the day.

Purifying Lemony Ginger Drink

Lemon can help neutralize the free radicals that invade your body, while ginger has anti-oxidant properties that can help your digestive system. Together, they can be a potent combination in battling the nasty invaders, and purify your body from harmful elements.

You will need:

2 lemons

1 small cucumber

Half inch ginger

1/2 cup mint leaves

2 quarts water

1 cup crushed ice

Here's how:

Wash all your ingredients and drain excess water. Peel your cucumber and ginger. Slice your cucumber, grate your ginger, and crush your mint leaves lightly. Line your ingredients at the bottom of your pitcher and muddle for a bit. Add your crushed ice and water and infuse for at least four hours in your refrigerator.

You can refill your pitcher up to five times, or until your ingredients become bland. You can use the same ingredients throughout the day.

Coco Loco Over Berries

The coconut water and berries combination is probably one of the most refreshing drinks that you will encounter. Berries have anti-cancer agents and can help preserve the youthful look of your skin. Coconut water has more potassium than four bananas combined, is low in calories, and has no cholesterol.

You will need:

1 cup raspberries

1 cup blackberries

1 liter coconut water

1 quart water

1 cup crushed ice

Here's how:

Wash your ingredients thoroughly and drain the excess water. Leave most of your berries as whole, and cut some berries in half. Line your ingredients at the bottom of your pitcher, and muddle them a little. Pour your coconut water and muddle some more before adding crushed ice and one quart water. You can opt to use 2 liters of coconut water instead of adding plain water.

Infuse for four hours in your refrigerator before serving.

Although water is enough to flush the toxins out of your body, the vitamins and other nutrients that the fruits and herbs impart in the water made these drinks even more effective.

Chapter 4 - Invigorating and Hydrating Water Recipes

The recipes for fruit infused water in this chapter provide your body with an energizing effect that can keep you going throughout the day. You will feel fresh, hydrated, and full of energy all day.

Minty Raspberry and Lime Water

The lime and raspberry combination gives a wonderful flavor blend. The addition of mint makes this drink a refreshing thirst quencher that will have you craving for more.

You will need:

2 cups raspberries

1 lime

Half cup of mint

2 quarts water

1 cup crushed ice

Here's how:

Wash your ingredients thoroughly and drain. Cut your lime into thin slices. Mash your raspberries lightly, just enough to release their intense flavor. Crush your mint leaves and line all your ingredients at the bottom of your pitcher. Muddle your ingredients a little then add your crushed ice and water. Infuse for at least three hours in the refrigerator before drinking.

You can refill your pitcher and use the same ingredients in the pitcher up to five times. Always keep in mind to refill your pitcher when it is half empty, and not totally empty.

Minty Water with Cherry and Cucumber

This drink has different flavor intensities, depending on the kind of cherry that you use. You will be able to feel its refreshing hydrating power after drinking just one glass.

You will need:

1 cup fresh cherries (pitted)

1 small to medium sized cucumber

Half cup of mint

2 quarts water

1 cup crushed ice

Here's how:

Carefully wash your ingredients and make sure to clean them thoroughly. Peel your cucumber and slice it thinly. Crush the mint leaves and lightly mash the cherries. Put your ingredients at the bottom of your pitcher and muddle for a bit. Add your crushed ice and pour water over your ingredients. Infuse for three to four hours in your refrigerator before serving.

You can refill your pitcher up to four times, or if your ingredients no longer give the kind of intensity in flavor that you want.

Tangy Kiwi Drink

If you want a simple yet tangy fruit infused water, then this recipe is for you.

You will need:

4 ripe kiwis

2 quarts water

1 cup crushed ice

Here's how:

Wash your kiwis and slice them thinly. Line your kiwi slices at the bottom of your pitcher. Add crushed ice and muddle a little. Pour water over it, and infuse for three to five hours in your refrigerator before serving. You can add kiwi slices to your glass as garnishing.

You can also crush your kiwis first to release a more intense flavor before putting your ingredients in the pitcher. Add your crushed ice and muddle it for a bit before pouring your water over. Infuse for two to three hours in your refrigerator. Garnish your glass with some kiwi slices, and you can strain the seeds as you pour your kiwi water drink in a glass. Serve and enjoy.

Refreshing Honeydew and Strawberry Water

If you want to taste a different kind of fruit juice without adding sugar, then you have got to sample this drink.

You will need:

1 cup honeydew (washed and cubed)

2 cups strawberries (washed and sliced)

2 quarts water

1 cup crushed ice

Here's how:

Line your fruits at the bottom of your pitcher and muddle a little. Add crushed ice and water. Infuse for four hours in your refrigerator before serving.

You can also use melon or cantaloupe instead of honeydew.

Berries Explosion

This recipe is like a gathering of berries that gives you a flavor explosion, and will have you yearning for more.

You will need:

1/2 cup strawberries

1/2 cup blueberries

1/2 cup blackberries

2 quarts water

1 cup crushed ice

Here's how:

Wash the berries and slice them in quarters. Line them at the bottom of your pitcher and mash them lightly (just enough to release more flavors) with your muddler. Add crush ice and water over your ingredients. Infuse for four hours or overnight to get a more explosive flavor. Serve and enjoy.

The hydrating and energizing drinks in this chapter can help you a lot in replenishing your energy and keeping your body hydrated during intense workouts, or if you need to finish a certain chore without delay.

Chapter 5 - Weight Loss Aid Recipes

The recipes for fruit infused water in this chapter can help you boost your metabolism, and lose weight. Although all recipes of fruit infused water can provide such benefits, the recipes in this chapter can provide especially good benefits regarding weight loss and metabolism.

Tangerine and Strawberry Medley

The beauty of this drink is that it's easy to make, refreshing, delicious, and economical. You can easily gather the ingredients and prepare it anytime of the day.

You will need:

1 cup strawberries (sliced)

1 tangerine (sliced)

2 quarts water

1 cup crushed ice

Here's how:

Put all of your ingredients in the pitcher and mash them a bit using your wooden spoon or muddler. The mashing will help release the flavors of the fruits. Add crushed ice and stir a little before adding your water over the ingredients. Infuse for four hours in your refrigerator before serving.

Blueberry and Pineapple Jumble

This drink is a mixture of blueberry and pineapple, and will give you an instant boost in the morning. The rich color of blueberries and the sweetness of pineapple are just perfect to get you going.

You will need:

1 cup blueberries (quartered)

1 cup pineapple (cubed)

2 quarts water

1 cup crushed ice

Here's how:

Line your fruits at the bottom of your pitcher. Muddle a little with a bit of mashing action. Add your crushed ice and water. Stir and infuse for four hours in your refrigerator. Serve and enjoy.

Grapefruit and Sage Combo

Grapefruit can reduce the insulin levels in your body which can lead to weight loss. There are dieters who feast on grapefruit to help them lose excess pounds. The catch is that grapefruit can interact with some medications, and if you are under medication, it is best to consult your doctor first before adding this fruit to your meal. Sage is also an effective ingredient for weight loss, and it can also help improve the condition of your hair.

You will need:

2 cups grapefruit (mashed)

3 tsp sage (ground)

2 quarts water

1 cup crushed ice

Here's how:

Put all your ingredients inside your pitcher. Add crushed ice and muddle a little before adding water over the ingredients. Stir once, and infuse for four hours in your refrigerator before serving.

Pomegranate in Blue

Pomegranate and blueberries are rich in antioxidants. This drink will have very high levels of antioxidants, especially if you mash the ingredients lightly before adding the water over the ingredients.

You will need:

1 pomegranate

2 cups blueberries

2 quarts water

1 cup crushed ice

Here's how:

You can remove the seeds of pomegranate, and submerge the slices of the fruit in a bowl of water. Strain the seeds and put them in your pitcher. Add your blueberries. Muddle the ingredients a little. Add crushed ice and water over the ingredients. Infuse for four hours in the refrigerator before you pour some in your glass and enjoy.

Zesty Ginger and Pear Twist

Pears are among the so called versatile fruits that you can do almost anything with. Pears can also reduce cholesterol levels, and help a person trying to lose weight. Combining pears with ginger equals one zesty and delightful drink that you will surely enjoy.

You will need:

2 pears (sliced)

1/4 cup ginger (peeled and sliced)

2 quarts water

1 cup crushed ice

Here's how:

Put everything in your pitcher. Mash the ingredients with your muddler. Add crushed ice and water. Infuse for one to two hours at room temperature and another four hours in your refrigerator. Strain to get clear water before serving. You can garnish your glass with pear and ginger slices.

Even if you are not trying to lose weight or looking for ways to achieve better looking skin, you can still choose to prepare any of the infused water recipes in this book. You don't need a specific goal to drink fruit infused water – just drink it because it is good for your body, because you need to reach your required amount of water, and because it's delicious.

Make it a habit to drink fruit infused water everyday and make it a point to reach your target water intake in a day to keep the bugs away.

Conclusion

Thank you again for downloading this book!

I hope this book was able to help you learn more about infused water, and all of the benefits it has to offer. It should not be all that difficult for you to make the healthy switch.

All the ingredients you need are available at your local produce market. The only other ingredients that you absolutely need, are your willingness to give it a try, and the willpower to resist sugary and artificially flavored drinks.

The next step is to put this information to use, and begin creating your own delicious infused water!

Finally, if you enjoyed this book, please take the time to share your thoughts and post a review on Amazon. It'd be greatly appreciated!

Thank you and good luck!

www.ingramcontent.com/pod-product-compliance
Lightning Source LLC
LaVergne TN
LVHW021744060526
838200LV00052B/3459